NEW ZEALAND HEADING DOG

The Complete Handbook On How To Raising And Caring For New Zealand Heading Dog

CHAD BRUNO

Table of Contents

Introductory

The term "New Zealand heading dog" normally refers to a breed of herding dog that is often seen in New Zealand. Their herding skills make them useful for tending to livestock, especially sheep. Their method of herding entails bending low and utilizing the dog's body and gaze to steer livestock, especially sheep, in the right direction, earning them the nickname "heading dogs."

• New Zealand heading dogs are highly regarded for their brains, speed, and independence in challenging environments. They are exceptionally talented at moving livestock and are coveted by farmers and ranchers for their herding ability.

While the word "heading dog" may have a different connotation in other countries, in New Zealand it is most often associated with the herding dogs used to herd sheep and cattle. These dogs are vital to New Zealand's agricultural sector.

CHAPTER ONE
Specifications and Types

There are various breeds that are commonly linked with New Zealand heading dogs, or heading dogs in general, since they share specific features. Some of the most common traits and breeds of heading dogs are as follows:

1. Breeding heading dogs with a high herding instinct is a common practice. They have an innate talent for herding livestock, which they express by crouching, stalking, and directing the animals with their eyes and body language.

2. Heading dogs have a reputation for being exceptionally bright. They have the ability to quickly appraise situations, make decisions, and follow directions.

3. Agility: These canines are swift on their feet and have excellent agility. They need quick reflexes and agility to get their work done on farms and ranches, where the terrain can be rough and difficult at times.

4. Heading dogs have great stamina, which allows them to herd sheep for lengthy periods of time and cover enormous regions.

5. They are quite amenable to training and quickly pick up on cues given to them. Because of this, they are excellent at tending to cattle and listening to their human handlers.

Some popular types of heading dogs are as follows:

1. One of the most well-known and popular breeds of heading dog is the Border Collie. They have a reputation for being excellent herders, are quite bright, and full of energy.

2. The history of the Australian Shepherd may be traced back to the

United States, despite the dog's name. As a result of their intelligence and agility, they are also effective herding dogs.

3. Blue Heelers and Queensland Heelers are two common names for the Australian Cattle Dog, which is commonly used as a heading dog for herding cattle. They tend their flocks with strength, loyalty, and skill.

4. The Australian Kelpie is another breed commonly used to herd sheep and other livestock. Their hard ethic and quickness are legendary.

5. Although not a "crouching and stalking" type of heading dog, the New Zealand Huntaway is a herding breed commonly used to move cattle around in that country. They herd animals by barking at them.

It's worth noting that "heading dog" and "herding dog" may have various connotations and be used to refer to different breeds of dogs depending on where you live. These dogs are highly prized in the agricultural and ranching communities because to their natural herding instincts and skill sets.

How to Take Good Care of Your Dog

Caring for your dog is of essential importance for various reasons. Dogs are more than just animals kept as pets; they are true members of the family. Their health, happiness, and longevity, as well as your own, all depend on how well you care for them. Some of the most important reasons to take good care of your dog are as follows:

1. For your dog's health and happiness, make sure he gets plenty of fresh water, gets out and plays regularly, and eats a balanced diet. This guarantees they keep up their physical health and may continue to fully participate in life.

2. Vaccinations, checkups, and preventative treatment (such as flea and tick control and heartworm prevention) administered at regular intervals by a veterinarian can help spot and treat potential health problems before they worsen.

3. In order to minimize destructive boredom in dogs, it is important to provide them with mental stimulation. Mental stimulation can be maintained through play, the provision of toys, and the performance of training tasks.

4. Dogs' mental health is important since they are pack animals that want affection and company. Maintaining their mental health requires consistent attention, affection, and instruction based on positive reinforcement.

5. Maintaining a clean and healthy dog is as simple as giving him a weekly wash, combing him, and cutting his nails. The presence of ticks and fleas on the skin can also be detected.

6. The welfare of your dog should always come first. This includes utilizing correct identification (such as tags and microchips), keeping them on a leash at all times, and keeping your home and yard secure.

7. A well-mannered and happy dog is the product of careful training and early socialization. You and your pet will develop a deeper connection if you do this.

8. Dog ownership requires a person to commit to a long-term responsibility. As they age and their needs alter, it is our responsibility to continue meeting those needs.

9. The ethical and legal responsibilities of pet ownership include compliance with local ordinances requiring registration, vaccinations, and the use of a leash. We have an ethical obligation to treat all animals humanely.

10. Dogs are great companions and friends, and they may help bolster the mental and emotional health of their human families. If properly cared for, they can continue performing this function for a long time.

11. Education and Bonding: Taking the time to learn about your dog's breed, special needs, and behavior will help you create a better bond and give more tailored care.

12. Taking good care of your dog has ramifications for public health. Well-cared-for dogs are less likely to spread disease, and dogs owned by responsible people are less likely to cause problems for neighbors.

Taking good care of your dog is a joyful and enriching experience that pays off in the form of a stronger bond between you and your pet. The joy and companionship a well-cared-for dog can bring is priceless, but the time, energy, and resources required to give one are substantial.

CHAPTER TWO
Getting a Good Heading Dog in New Zealand

Choosing the perfect New Zealand heading dog, or herding dog in general, is a big deal that requires a lot of thought. You should make sure that your lifestyle and the requirements of these pets match up. Follow these instructions to pick the perfect New Zealand heading dog:

1. Do your homework: To begin, read up on the breed and its typical traits. Learn the characteristics, levels of activity, and personalities of New Zealand heading dogs. Think about how well their natural herding tendencies align with your own.

2. Think About Your Way of Life, Living Arrangement, and Physical Activity Level. High-energy heading dogs need an owner who can keep up with them physically and mentally. You really shouldn't get this breed if you're a couch potato.

3. Think About Your Background Most heading dogs benefit from having experienced dog owners who know how to train and control them. You should either have experience working with dogs already or be willing to put in some time and effort to train a heading dog if this is your first pet.

4. A New Zealand heading dog may be the best option if you live on a farm or ranch and require a dog for herding animals. They're bred specifically for herding and are very good at it.

5. Think on whether you want a New Zealand heading dog primarily as a companion or a working partner for sheep. These dogs can make wonderful friends, but they may still need outlets for their herding impulses.

**6.   Socialization: **Proper socialization is vital. If you want your New Zealand heading dog to grow up socially and act well, you should start socializing it early with a wide range of people, animals, and settings.

7. Choose between buying a dog from a reputable breeder or adopting a dog from a rescue group. Both choices offer significant benefits, but it's more important that the dog is healthy and well-cared for once you bring it home.

8. When purchasing a puppy from a breeder, it is important to meet both of the puppy's parents. This might tell you a lot about the dog's personality and behavior in the future.

9. Make sure the breeder you choose does health and genetic testing to eliminate or at least greatly lower the likelihood of heritable health problems. Although New Zealand heading dogs have a strong genetic foundation, occasionally they might develop health issues.

10. Be ready to put in some serious time and effort into training and obedience. Because of their intelligence, heading dogs require formal training to become obedient pets.

11. Make sure you have enough room for physical activity and mental stimulation. Having a yard that is fenced in safely is crucial.

12. Realize that training a herding dog is a lengthy process that takes patience and dedication. Be ready to invest in their education and work with them continuously.

Careful deliberation and planning are needed to select the ideal New Zealand heading dog. You can select a dog that will suit your needs and make a fantastic addition to your family or farm if you take the time to learn about the breed and evaluate your own lifestyle and commitment level.

Don't Leave New Zealand without Your Heading Dog

Bringing your New Zealand-bound dog home is a milestone in your canine ownership journey, filled with excitement and responsibility. It's crucial to make things easy on yourself and your new friend. Bringing Your New Zealand Heading Dog Home is Easy If You Follow These Steps

Earlier than bringing your dog inside:

1. Ensure the safety of your dog by dog-proofing your home by fastening or removing any items your dog could chew on, ingest, or escape from. This encompasses anything from potentially poisonous flora and chemicals to small, easily accessible things.

2. Acquire Necessary Items: Invest in a crate (if wanted), food and water dishes, high-quality dog food, a leash and collar, tags, a comfy bed, toys, and grooming tools.

3. Create a Safe Space: Designate a separate space or room where your dog can retire to when they need seclusion or rest. This area needs to feel safe and welcoming.

Transporting Your Dog:

1. Take all necessary precautions to ensure your dog's safe and comfortable travel to your house. The dog's breeder, from whom you'll be acquiring him or her, may offer advice on this matter.

2. When you get home, take baby steps in acclimating your dog to his or her new surroundings. Let them check out one area at a time, but keep a tight eye on them as they do so.

3. For the first few days, continue the feeding schedule set by the breeder or former owner. If changing your diet is necessary, do so gradually. Always have clean water on hand.

4. Dogs do well with regular routines. Incorporate training and playing into your pet's daily routine. They like the reliability.

5. Education and Socialization: Educate and integrate young. Basic obedience training and pleasant social contacts are vital for your dog's development.

6. Always keep an eye on your dog, but especially for the first two weeks. This ensures their safe adaptation to their new environment and reduces the likelihood of accidents.

7. Offer solace and reassurance to the one in need. Your dog may be feeling nervous or uncertain about their new environment; please be patient with them. Invest in pleasant interactions and time together to build a strong bond.

8. Dogs should always wear identification tags with your contact information, and microchipping is another option for both safety and identification in case they become lost. If they become lost, this information will be vital.

Condition of the body:

1. Make an Appointment with the Vet: Have your dog checked up by the vet soon after you bring it home. This is necessary so that we may discuss immunizations, preventative care, and spaying/neutering from a starting point of their current health.

2. Prevention of Fleas, Ticks, and Worms Have a talk with your vet about starting preventative measures against fleas, ticks, and worms.

3. Do not forget to document your dog's health history and vaccines.

Physical Health:

1. Spend time with your dog and show him or her lots of affection. A dog's emotional health depends on the strength of the link its owner has with it.

2. New Zealand heading dogs are high-energy pets that need regular playtime and mental stimulation. To maintain a healthy state of mind and disposition, make sure they get plenty of physical activity and mental challenge.

Keep in mind that every dog is different and the adjustment process could take some time. You may help your New Zealand heading dog adjust and grow in its new home by being patient and providing it with a secure, caring environment.

CHAPTER THREE
Food and Nourishment

The health and happiness of your New Zealand heading dog depends on your attention to its diet and feeding routine. Because of their high energy levels, it is essential to feed these dogs a healthy, well-rounded diet. Nutritional and feeding recommendations for your New Zealand heading dog are as follows:

1. Before making any major dietary changes to your dog, it is recommended that you speak with your veterinarian. They'll be able to tailor their advice to your dog based on factors including his or her age, size, degree of exercise, and health.

2. Grade Commercial Dog Food Select a commercial dog food of a high grade. Try to find products where the first ingredient is a meat, poultry, or fish protein source. Your dog will get all the nutrients it needs from high-quality dog food.

3. Consider the Life Stage: Dogs have diverse nutritional requirements at distinct life stages. It's important to feed your dog a formula designed for his or her age, whether it's a puppy, adult, or senior.

4. Because of their high activity levels, New Zealand heading dogs need a diet rich in protein. Muscle growth and repair rely heavily on protein.

5. Fat: You need some fat to keep going, and it helps your skin and hair look good, too. Active dogs need dog food with higher fat content.

6. Dogs don't require a high-carb diet, but the energy they provide is worth considering. Include brown rice, oats, and sweet potatoes in your diet for their whole grains.

7. Feed your dog a quantity that is reasonable for its age, size, and degree of exercise. The health risks associated with obesity are real, and they can be exacerbated by overeating.

8. Set a regular eating routine, consisting of at least two meals per day. Do not leave food out all day, as this can encourage snacking and lead to weight gain.

9. Provide your dog with plenty of fresh, clean water at all times. Active dogs, in particular, need to drink a lot of water.

10. Chocolate, grapes, raisins, onions, garlic, and some artificial sweeteners are just some of the human delicacies that can be deadly to dogs. Make sure your dog has no way of getting at these items.

11. Treats and Snacks: Cut back on the quantity. Make sure the treats you use for training or occasional rewards are safe for dogs.

12. Taking your dog in for examinations at the vet on a regular basis will allow you to keep tabs on his or her weight and health. If necessary, they might also suggest changes to your diet.

13. If your pet has allergies, sensitivities, or a medical condition, your doctor may suggest a special diet. Listen carefully to their advice.

14. Pay Attention to Your Dog's Condition Always be aware of how your dog's physique looks. Without a significant amount of fat, your ribs should be easily palpable. Talk to your vet if you're unsure of their size.

Whether your New Zealand heading dog is working on a farm or just being your buddy, they need a healthy, well-balanced food to thrive. Tailor their nutrition to their particular needs, and be vigilant to any changes in their health, activity level, or food preferences as they mature.

Hygiene and Medical Care

New Zealand heading dogs require regular grooming and veterinary treatment. Maintaining your dog's health, comfort, and happiness can be accomplished with regular grooming and veterinary care. The following are recommendations for the care and maintenance of your New Zealand heading dog:

Grooming:

1. The coat of a New Zealand heading dog is normally short to medium in length and sheds at specific times of the year. Brushing their coat on a regular basis helps eliminate dead hair, avoids mats, and maintains the coat clean. At the very least, brush your dog once a week, and more often if you live in a high-shedding area.

2. Dogs should be washed when they are dirty or smelly, but otherwise just as needed. Use a gentle dog wash and rinse gently to get rid of any soap.

3. Keep your dog's nails at a manageable length to prevent injury and discomfort. Regular nail trimming is vital, especially for dogs with high activity levels.

4. Care for your dog's ears by keeping a regular check for debris, excess wax, or infection. If necessary, use ear cleaning solution designed for dogs and a soft cloth to clean their ears.

5. Proper Dental Hygiene Is Crucial To Overall Health. To prevent plaque and tartar buildup, it is important to either brush your dog's teeth on a regular basis or provide dental chews and toys.

6. Care for the Eyes: Look for Discharge or Irritation in Your

Dog's Eyes. Wipe away any discharge with a wet cloth and visit your vet if the issue persists.

Healthcare:

1. When it comes to immunizations, follow your vet's advice and make sure your dog is up to date. Rabies and distemper vaccines are examples of core immunizations.

2. Controlling Parasites: Get Rid of Them! Regular deworming and treatments for parasites like fleas and ticks are part of this. To find out what products are best for your dog and your location, go to your vet.

3. Talk to your veterinarian about spaying or neutering your pet. The timing of this surgery, which might prevent undesired litters and provide some health benefits, may vary based on your dog's age and other factors.

4. Visiting the vet regularly is essential for keeping an eye on your pet's health. Any potential health problems can be identified and treated early with the help of these checkups.

5. New Zealand heading dogs are known to be extremely energetic, which can make them vulnerable to overuse injuries. Ensure kids get appropriate exercise while also being wary of potential strains or injuries.

6. Do your best to keep your dog at a healthy weight. Many health issues are linked to obesity. If you want to know how much your dog should weigh, it's best to ask your vet.

7. In terms of nutrition, it's important to give your dog a food tailored to its needs. Talk to your vet about any issues or preferences you have regarding your pet's nutrition.

8. Consider the possibility that your dog has food or environmental sensitivity. Consult your vet for advice if you observe symptoms of allergies, including as skin irritations or gastrointestinal problems.

9. Have a plan in place in case of an emergency. Having a basic pet first-aid kit on hand and knowing the location of the nearest 24-hour veterinarian clinic are also necessary.

10. Training and Behavioral Problems should be dealt with immediately, and if necessary, specialized training should be considered. In the same way that physical health is crucial, so too is mental health.

You may help your New Zealand heading dog have a long, healthy, and happy life by adopting certain habits for grooming and medical care. Consistent veterinary checkups and preventative treatment are crucial for identifying and treating health issues in their earliest, most treatable stages.

CHAPTER FOUR
Instruction in Simple Commands and Obedience

Obedience and command training are crucial to the health, happiness, and peace of mind of your New Zealand heading dog. Because of their high IQ and boundless energy, these dogs take to training quite quickly. To help you educate your New Zealand heading dog, here are some fundamental instructions and pointers:

1. Sit:

• Put the dog on a leash first.

• Raise a reward high above their head.

• The "Sit" order is accompanied by a backward and slightly upward motion of the treat.

Dogs are naturally obedient, so when they smell a treat, they should sit. Give them the treat and some compliments when they do.

2. Stay:

• The first step is to get your dog to sit.

Show your open hand like a stop sign and say "Stay" as you take a backwards step.

• Take a break, and then come back to your dog.

• Offer a treat and some words of appreciation if they stay sitting. As they get better, gradually extend the time and distance.

3. Remember (Come)

Put the dog on a leash first.

• Crouch down and open your arms while shouting "Come" in an enticing tone.

• As soon as your dog comes over to you, give them a treat and some compliments.

• Practice this in several situations and progressively increase the distance between you and your dog.

4. Down:

The first step is to get your dog to sit.

• Say "Down" while you lower a goodie near their nose and watch them respond positively.

You should praise and treat your dog when it follows the goodie to the floor and lays down.

5. Put It Away:

• Present your dog with a reward while keeping your hand closed.

To prevent your dog from stealing the treat, close your palm and firmly command, "Leave it."

• Hold off rewarding your dog until he or she loses interest in the treat.

• Acknowledge their effort and give them a special reward.

6. Walking on a leash (or a heel):

Put the dog on a leash first.

• Keep the leash loose and have your dog stroll by your left side.

Words like "Heel" can be used as verbal cues to keep your dog close by.

If your dog remains in the desired position, praise him or her.

7. Don't Leap:

• Teach your dog not to jump on people by ignoring them when they do it and shouting "No" or "Off."

• Give your dog lots of attention and praise when it remains on the ground with all four paws.

Hints for Training:

• Use positive reinforcement: Reward-based training using treats, praise, and affection is the most effective way for heading dogs.

- Train your dog frequently but briefly to keep him interested.

- Exert patience and constancy. Dogs learn via repetition, so practice constantly.

- Give a single, unambiguous instruction for each action.

- Practice in a variety of settings so that cues may be applied anywhere.

Avoid punishment-based approaches because they often result in defensiveness and hostility.

Training your dog to obey your commands is an ongoing process that must be maintained throughout the dog's life. New Zealand heading dogs are highly trainable and eager to please, making them ideal for specialized work on farms and ranches.

Physical Activity and Cognitive Enhancement

New Zealand heading dogs require a lot of exercise and mental activity. These canines are extremely lively and bright; they benefit much from mental and physical stimulation. Some suggestions on how to give your dog the physical and emotional stimulation it needs:

Exercise:

1. Daily Exercise: Daily exercise is a must for New Zealand heading dogs. Get at least 60–90 minutes of exercise every day, spread up over several sessions if necessary.

2. The best way to get rid of their boundless energy is to take them for regular walks, runs, and excursions. You should think about signing them up for dog sports or classes, since they would do very well in situations requiring agility and obedience.

3. Heading dogs are known to like in games of fetch. They can enjoy vigorous games of catch or frisbee with a ball.

4. Hiking & Outdoor Activities: Take your dog on hiking and outdoor excursions. They get a kick out of experiencing novel settings and difficulties.

5. If you own a farm or livestock, your dog will be invaluable for herding. They get to work out while doing something that gives them purpose.

6. Many working dogs consider swimming and water retrieval to be among their favorite pastimes. Make sure your dog is used to being around water and that the place is secure.

7. Off-Leash Play: Give your dog a chance to go about and play without being restrained by a leash in a safe, gated area.

Stimulating the Mind:

1. Consistent training sessions are a great method to keep the mind active. Show them some new tricks and make sure they know the old ones.

2. Challenge your dog's intelligence with puzzle toys and interactive feeders.

3. Play a game of hide-and-seek with your dog by hiding their favorite treats or toys.

4. Use your dog's keen sense of smell to your advantage with some scent work.

5. To keep your dog interested in his or her toys, rotate them on a regular basis. Toys, such as chew toys and puzzle toys, should be made available.

6. To ensure that your dog always has well-honed social abilities, it is important to socialize it on a regular basis.

7. If you have a farm, your dog will love getting to exercise his or her herding instincts by helping out with the daily chores.

8. Obstacle Courses: Set up obstacle courses or agility equipment in your yard for your dog to navigate.

9. Mental Exercises: Keep your dog's mind active by training it to tell the difference between different things or complete more difficult activities.

10. Play and cuddle with your dog and give him lots of love. They adore bonding with their owners.

Keeping your New Zealand heading dog mentally stimulated can be just as taxing as physically exercising it. A dog that has had plenty of exercise is a tired dog. Fulfilling their need for stimulation and preventing boredom, which can lead to behavioral problems, can be aided by giving both physical activity and mental challenges. It also helps you and your dog become closer to one another.

CHAPTER FIVE

Concerns Regarding Progeny

Breeding dogs is a huge responsibility and decision that should not be taken lightly. Several considerations must be made to guarantee the safety and well-being of the dogs involved in any breeding program. Whether you're raising New Zealand heading dogs or another breed, keep these things in mind:

1. Examining Your Health:

• Both the male and female canines should be subjected to comprehensive health checks and genetic testing for breed-specific and inherited disorders prior to mating.

Make sure the dogs are healthy and free of genetic disorders by consulting a veterinarian and a canine geneticist.

2. Temperament:

• The temperament of the male and female dog is equally important. Dogs with appealing and consistent personalities that also conform to the breed standard should be bred.

3. Expertise and Experience:

• Breeders that are serious about their craft will study the breed extensively to learn all they can about its history, health, and genetics.

• Knowledge and practice in canine care and training are prerequisites for breeding.

4. Breeding with Integrity and Responsibility:

• Breeding should be done with the welfare of the breed in mind, not for financial gain or for fun.

Maintain ethical breeding techniques by ensuring that puppies receive the care, socialization, and training they need.

5. Guidelines for Breeding:

• Only breed animals that meet specific standards for appearance, health, and demeanor.

• Aim to have puppies that improve the overall genetic makeup of the breed.

6. Parental Dogs' Age and Health:

• The male and female partner(s) must be in pristine health.

Do not breed puppies from young or old dogs. The best time to start breeding should be discussed with your veterinarian.

7. Permission to Breed and Restrictions:

• Take note of any restrictions on breeding dogs that may exist in your area. There are regulations and rules that must be followed in order to obtain a breeding license in some areas.

8. Meeting Compatible Partners:

• Choose male and female dogs that are good fits for each other in terms of health, temperament, and genetics.

For help in selecting compatible partners, you should reach out to breed clubs, registries, and seasoned breeders.

9. Variation in genes:

• Protect the breed's genetic variety to lower the prevalence of heritable diseases.

• Inbreeding should be avoided at all costs; it raises the risk of transmitting genes that cause disease.

10. Domestic Setting:

• Provide a clean, healthy, and secure home environment for the breeding dogs and puppies, and make sure they get plenty of attention, exercise, and socialization.

11. Adoption of a Dog:

• Have a plan for finding good homes for your puppies. Vet would-be pet owners to make sure they can give the animal the attention it deserves.

12. Maintaining Accurate Records

• Keep meticulous medical, breeding, and progeny records for each dog.

- This data is crucial for genealogical and medical record keeping.

13. Seek Advice from a Guide:

• If you're new to breeding, it's a good idea to find an experienced person to help you along the way.

Always put the health and happiness of the dogs and the puppies first, as breeding is a lifelong commitment. It is crucial to put the breed's well-being first, to use only ethical breeding methods, and to follow all relevant rules and regulations. Breeding dogs responsibly is a big responsibility that requires a lot of time and research as well as a serious dedication to the dogs and the breed as a whole.

Care for the Elderly and the Dying

It's crucial to give your aging New Zealand heading dog the love and attention it needs to live out its final days in peace and comfort. Some things to think about as you age and approach the end of life are listed below.

1. Checkups with the Vet:

• Various health problems become more common in senior dogs. The importance of having your pet examined by a veterinarian regularly increases so that any health issues can be caught early and treated.

2. Modified Food Plan:

• To meet your dog's evolving nutritional requirements, discuss dietary changes with your vet. Formulas designed specifically for senior dogs are an option.

3. Physical Movement:

• Your aging dog may not have the same boundless enthusiasm as they did when they were younger, but they still need regular, gentle exercise to keep them mobile and slim. Adjust the intensity and duration of exercise to suit their age and health.

4. Relaxation and Security:

• Improve your home so that an elderly dog can live there in peace and security. There should be easy access to food and water, as well as comfortable bedding.

5. Treatment Methods for Discomfort:

• Talk to your vet about medications and pain management options for your dog if they suffer from age-related health problems **like arthritis.**

6. Care for Your Teeth:

• Maintain regular dental checkups to avoid painful dental issues that can signal underlying health problems.

7. Mental Wellness:

• Dementia-like cognitive decline is common in geriatric dogs. Give them something to think about, like a puzzle or an activity toy.

8. Making a Final Choice:

• As your dog nears the end of their life, you may be forced to make some tough choices. For advice on end-of-life care, pain management, and palliative treatment options, talk to your vet.

9. Life satisfaction:

• Maintain a consistent evaluation of your dog's well-being. Do they hurt more than they feel good? It may be necessary to consider euthanasia when your dog's quality of life declines significantly.

10. Assistance with Feelings:

• Shower your senior dog with affection, time, and care. Comfort them in their old age by spending time with them and showing affection.

11. Hospice Treatment:

• Hospice care can help make sure your dog is as comfortable and happy as possible if you decide against euthanizing them when their health declines.

12. Euthanasia:

• If your dog's quality of life has been drastically reduced due to illness or injury, it is the kind and humane thing to do to put an end to its suffering. Your vet will be able to help you through this.

13. Grief Counseling:

• Realize that dealing with the death of a pet can be difficult emotionally. If you need help adjusting to your loss, don't hesitate to reach out for comfort from those close to you.

You can show your love for your aging New Zealand heading dog by giving it the best possible end-of-life care. Make decisions that respect their wishes for their final days with the same care and consideration you gave them throughout their lives.

Conclusion

Providing for the physical, mental, and emotional needs of a New Zealand heading dog throughout its life is a rewarding experience. Dog ownership is a rewarding and lifelong commitment that includes picking the right dog and providing it with a healthy diet, regular exercise, a clean environment, and veterinary care.

A well-mannered and happy companion or working dog can only be achieved through proper training and socialization. They need regular physical activity and mental challenges to thrive.

Providing compassionate end-of-life care is a final act of love and responsibility, and it becomes increasingly important as your dog ages and your needs change.

The bond you share with your New Zealand heading dog is unique, and with the right amount of love and care, it can be a wonderful experience for both of you.

THE END